Medical Planner for Patients

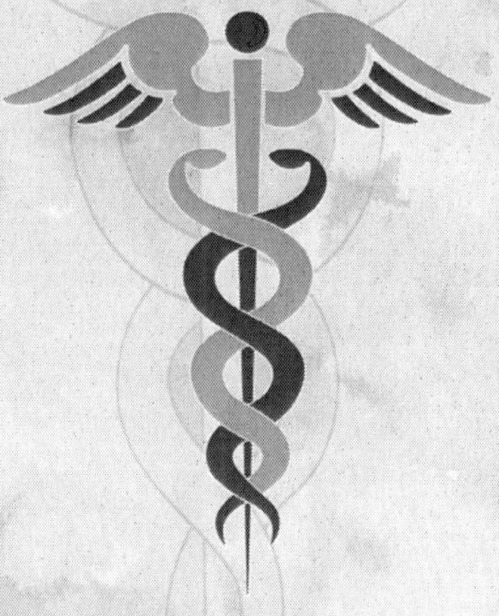

Mary Susan Carey

Medical Planner for Patients

Mary Susan Carey

Published by Angel Journal and Books,

Burlington, ON, Canada

First Edition: First Printing

Disclaimer: This material is for educational and self-help purposes only. It is not intended to diagnose, prescribe, treat, or cure any disease or mental condition. You are advised to consult appropriate health care providers on any matter concerning your physical, emotional and mental health.

This material is designed to work in consultation with your health care providers.

ISBN: 978-1-9992131-2-1

This Journal Belongs to:

____

Address:

____

____

Phone:

____

Email:

____

The Intent of this Journal

When serious illness is diagnosed, or chronic health conditions require constant support and medical guidance, it is very common to feel overwhelmed, confused, and even hopelessly disempowered.

This Planner is designed to help you keep better track of appointments and doctors' visits. It becomes quite difficult when you are a senior in age or the stress of the event seems to bring on brain freeze!

Writing everything down in one place can take a load off your mind. This plannr is designed to support you in this way. Everything can be recorded here for your handy reference. Take it with you to appointments and have your questions prepared for discussions with your doctors and health care providers.

If desired, glue an envelope inside the front or back cover to tuck reports and other loose papers into. Having everything in one place can support you and help you feel more focused during a very stressful time.

We are glad you have purchased this journal. We hope that it helps you through your treatments and that you improve or recover your health.

Doctors Addresses and Phone Numbers

Name Specialty	Address	Phone

Test Results

Test	Date	Result

Medication Tracker

Start Date	End Date	Medicine	Dosage	When to Take	Side Effects

January

Sun	Mon	Tue	Wed	Thu	Fri	Sat

Notes

February

Sun	Mon	Tue	Wed	Thu	Fri	Sat

Notes

March

Sun	Mon	Tue	Wed	Thu	Fri	Sat

Notes

April

Sun	Mon	Tue	Wed	Thu	Fri	Sat

Notes

May

Sun	Mon	Tue	Wed	Thu	Fri	Sat

Notes

June

Sun	Mon	Tue	Wed	Thu	Fri	Sat

Notes

July

Sun	Mon	Tue	Wed	Thu	Fri	Sat

Notes

August

Sun	Mon	Tue	Wed	Thu	Fri	Sat

Notes

September

Sun	Mon	Tue	Wed	Thu	Fri	Sat

Notes

October

Sun	Mon	Tue	Wed	Thu	Fri	Sat

Notes

November

Sun	Mon	Tue	Wed	Thu	Fri	Sat

Notes

December

Sun	Mon	Tue	Wed	Thu	Fri	Sat

Notes

Date: *My Issues to Discuss Today*

Patient Doctor Discussion Notes

My Issues to Discuss Today Date:

Patient Doctor Discussion Notes

Date: My Issues to Discuss Today

Patient Doctor Discussion Notes

My Issues to Discuss Today Date:

Patient Doctor Discussion Notes

Date: *My Issues to Discuss Today*

Patient Doctor Discussion Notes

My Issues to Discuss Today Date:

Patient Doctor Discussion Notes

Symptoms Tracker

Date	Time	Symptoms	Mild	Moderate	Severe
			☐	☐	☐
			☐	☐	☐
			☐	☐	☐
			☐	☐	☐
			☐	☐	☐
			☐	☐	☐
			☐	☐	☐
			☐	☐	☐
			☐	☐	☐
			☐	☐	☐
			☐	☐	☐
			☐	☐	☐
			☐	☐	☐
			☐	☐	☐

Symptoms Tracker

Date	Time	Symptoms	Mild	Moderate	Severe
			☐	☐	☐
			☐	☐	☐
			☐	☐	☐
			☐	☐	☐
			☐	☐	☐
			☐	☐	☐
			☐	☐	☐
			☐	☐	☐
			☐	☐	☐
			☐	☐	☐
			☐	☐	☐
			☐	☐	☐
			☐	☐	☐
			☐	☐	☐

*Date:*________________

Date:________________

*Date:*________________

Date:________________

*Date:*________________

*Date:*________________

Resources

Contact Information

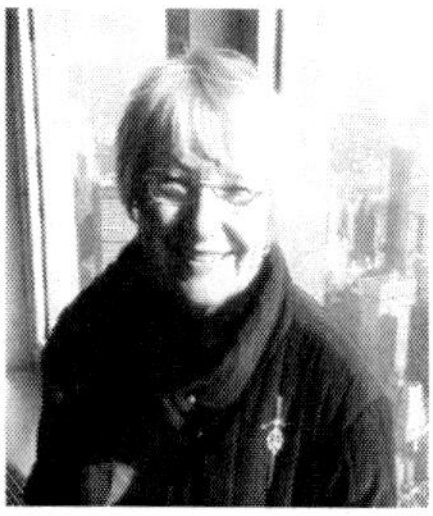

Mary Susan Carey

angeljournalbooks@gmail.com

angeljournal.com

amazon.com/author/angeljournal

Additional Journals and Planners

Angel Journal Guidance: Feel Powerful Be Guided

Angel Journal 44 Days of Daily Guidance

Garden Angel Journal and Planner

Golf Duffer's Diary from the 19th Hole

Magical Unicorns: A Diary and Doodle Book for Women

Magical Unicorns: A Diary and Doodle Book for Girls

Migraine Tracking Journal Version 2

Made in United States
North Haven, CT
04 November 2026

21765512R00023